The Autotoxic

Patient

AN EASIER HEALTH

Dr Timothy Glover

B Sc., D.C., D.O.

For

Jim Hoberg

CONTENTS

Introduction

Introduction

This book discusses how patients may undertake easy changes themselves, which I believe can lead to profound improvements in their health and importantly, their happiness.

Human beings are extraordinarily complex yet I consider if one looks at this complexity we are able to see a simplicity within that which is complex. What is simple may seem trivial or small yet can be very powerful and enable a patient to make critical changes so that the care of their health may become dramatically easier.

I am a practitioner of some twenty eight years clinical experience. It is that I have always strived to find better ways to help a patient improve more quickly and more easily. After attending over forty post graduate courses since completing university study, my feeling was that to continue to learn and improve my capability I had to develop work more so from my own thinking, from what science I could apply within my own practice.

And so this book contains in part a compilation of what I have developed within my practice and found to be somewhat unique or unusual, yet very powerful within the treatment of my patients.

In one sense over the last seven years as I have increased the bias of health care toward what a patient would do at home it has made the clinical treatment required far easier, much less time consuming and less expensive for the patient.

Having worked toward how to further improve as a clinician over the years, I feel very happy with what I am able to achieve in my treatment of a patient within the practice. My clinical approach or methodology is not within the scope of this book, though this will be covered in the coming text, CLINICAL THEORY, which has a bias more toward a practitioner's application.

I am now very aware of how exceptionally powerful often small and simple changes a patient can apply at home are and have been extraordinarily helpful.

So much of what I am able to do physically with a patient "in the office" as such I consider to be extremely effective, yet without changes in what a patient can do themselves, one does not work anywhere near as what I would require without the other.

With reference to this book's title "THE AUTOTOXIC PATIENT" I originally thought to use the term with regard to the idea that a patient may sustain an ongoing toxicity from retained segments of microbial nucleic acids (chapter 3). I feel though over time the term "AUTOTOXIC" also applies somewhat to toxicity acquired within a patient's home, work, their dietary habits and personal environment. That is as such that a patient is commonly suffering an ongoing internal and or external "automatic" toxicity. Addressing the above is so much of what I have found to be not only helpful with patients but in most cases an essential requirement. So often I believe that a patient is searching for a cure and yet they are living with the causes of their illness and that a greater part of the cure they seek is at home.

As a teenager I raced small boats, on occasion my father would take me to hear yachtsmen of some renown give talks upon various aspects with regard to sailing. I recall once saying to him, I wonder if these fellows will be any good (i.e. the speakers, and they were very good!, John Bertrand, Buddy Melges), my father's response was that if you pick up one thing that's useful, then you're in front!

I do hope that you the reader can find something that is useful, well, or more than that within this book, so that you may have a better, an easier health!

I have written this book, in a not so colloquial fashion. It is that I have attempted to write to a degree above what would be considered lay terms though in a fashion consistent with the language that I would use with a patient. This is in part deliberate in that I do like patients to have some understanding of their condition, their physiology and what it is that their treatment entails. Though some of the material may seem complex or unfamiliar I have retained that bias at least in part with a view not to oversimplify the work presented. With patients, they are able to ask questions so as to clarify aspects which may be difficult to understand, though as for the reader I would suggest either your practitioner or of course the internet is a useful tool.

Please note, the chapter, A Brief History may be of more interest to someone of a more technical persuasion or a practitioner. The chapter, "DNA", may be of some assistance to read toward an understanding of chapter 3. WHO'S GENES!

Overview

I feel that if I had read this book as young practitioner it may have seemed to me interesting and yet somewhat unusual. What I have come to see as very significant concepts and changes to assist a patient may seem somewhat surprising and out of the ordinary, in brief, as follows:

➢ Pernicious infection, that is the presence of chronic very low grade infection or infections, either systemically, i.e. throughout the body, or within particular parts, limbs, the skin, glands or internal organs.

➢ Accumulation of non self, genetic material within our own cells from infectious processes not only as would occur with a viral infection but as retained incomplete parts or segments of microbial DNA/RNA, i.e. nucleic acids or in other terms, non self "genes".

➢ Retention of old or oxidized or toxic fats and oils within the bile, hence a resultant limitation of our body's ability to remove used or unwanted fatty acids or to absorb from our food new fats and oils which are essential for normal metabolic functions.

➢ Metal toxicity or poisoning "so to speak" from for example jewellery, piercings, dental fillings, deodorant.

➢ Adverse or harmful sensory stimulation from jewellery especially earrings, piercings, rings, wrist watches or chains providing a source of dysfunction within not only our nervous system in a conventional sense but also across or within specific acupuncture meridians throughout the body.

➢ Lack of 'cycling' food in our diets i.e. eating or drinking the same food daily, or over months or years without a rest or change, leading in part to an accumulation of unusable material or waste within the body.

➤ The consideration of what could be termed an "Ancestral diet", that is, are we eating food which is suited to our genetic makeup and how the genetic constitution we have as individuals is able to allow us to adapt to the food we eat and do so within the environment in which we live?

➤ Toxicity within the home especially due to infectious matter e.g. fungus or bacteria that would live within old mattresses, pillows, books, clothes, furniture, carpet, air-conditioning.

➤ Toothpaste, that is, is fluoride good or bad? It is probably both! In finding a level of exposure or ingestion of fluoride which suits the patient it is I consider possible to affect a dramatic improvement in a patient's biochemistry and therefore of course, their level of health.

A Brief History

My undergraduate training was what I would prefer to call osteopathic, not dissimilar in length and subject matter to a medical course. The bias was much less toward pharmaceutical studies or surgical intervention and primarily with regard to treatment of the spine, peripheral joints and muscle function.

I believe my undergraduate course was a good one, very hard work and thorough. Early though in practice as a locum I felt that to a degree some of the promise as far as the effectiveness and range of treatment that I had expected while studying, though at times spectacularly successful was not as much up to what I desired as a practitioner.

As such as my interest to pursue postgraduate study was high. In addition to that I had and still do have a constant questioning within my own thinking very much aligned to "how does this work" "what is the essential problem with this patient", "if it works how can I do this better"?

In addition to formal courses my reading included aspects of Chinese medicine, homeopathic, ayuvedic and herbal medicines, lymphatic procedures, massage. I considered that the more I learnt the greater the range of tools available to apply and a better more integrated understanding to be had.

The most significant modality that I pursued was that of Applied Kinesiology which provided the concept of a link or links between a bony or joint fixation, muscle dysfunction and organic, glandular and metabolic functions. Not only did this study enable me to far more quickly improve joint function in a patient but also as an entrée into dealing with health problems other than those of primarily spinal or peripheral joint dysfunction.

In the late nineties a watershed series of clinical biochemistry courses presented by Christopher Astill Smith (Epigenetics Ltd), provided for me a far greater understanding of common ailments, their organic or metabolic character and the treatment of such conditions.

Following soon after the above series and what was a single course, one of the most useful that I have attended; presented by Dr Michael Allen (HealthBuilderS),which dealt with links and associations between a patient's posture, their muscle, metabolic and nervous system functions.

This course further augmented and was a progression upon aspects of what material I had found to be of value within the study of Applied Kinesiology. In addition, it enabled me to identify muscles that were "carrying" excess stimulation, or "normal" or having a deficiency of stimulus. The course presented a simple approach which provided to some extent a "window" into "looking at" and treating either "excess" activity or "deficient" activity within a variety of organic, glandular, neurological systems.

There above lays I believe a very useful modality to employ in examining a patient. Simple muscle stretch muscle reflex tests can be used to demonstrate some indications as to whether a patient, by way of analogy   has his or her "foot on the accelerator pedal and on the brake" at the same time, with respect to their muscle function for example. Just as with a motor car, a patient goes not so well with the brakes on while the accelerator pedal is pressed.

In identifying abnormal "offs" and "on's" within the nervous system, muscles, glands and organs one is then more able to instigate changes so as to develop more normal or healthier function. Also to enable improvement in patients that will be more profound and lasting.

In part as a result my practice has moved more toward improving health in a patient rather than simply treating or managing illness.

Importantly, one particular form or modality of testing as above does not negate the need for more conventional tests, orthopaedic, neurological, radiographic, laboratory tests or referrals to other practitioners.

There is no single form or approach to testing or examining a patient that is perfect and so using a collection of various methodology's, taking time so as to be thorough and especially to listen, to persistently re-examine, I believe is essential.

In utilising a multiplicity of tests one is able to look at or examine the body more so as a whole, that is to look at multiple systems, organs, glands, acupuncture meridians, neurotransmitters, functions as a whole and how they relate to one another, for example digestion or energy production. Not only does this enable the "seeing" of a broad "picture" yet also to be very specific as to what approaches to utilise with a patient.

In essence, the persistence with a diversity and thoroughness of testing or examination of patients has for me not only been of great assistance with clinical treatment yet so importantly enabling me to see causative factors within that persons "living" environment. Looking at a patient's home, work and personal environment and how those environments can be altered to greatly assist their health is very much part of the subject matter of this book.

WHO'S GENES?

Patients are not uncommonly told that the condition from which they suffer is genetic in origin or causation. This may well be true in many cases. In the field of genetics our "display" as a human being is a combination of phenotype and genotype. That is, what we are as a result of our environmental history i.e. diet, climate 'life' and our genetic expression. A few years ago I began to look into what I could do with regard to gene function especially to see if it were possible to produce some change which may be of a positive benefit to a patient.

At the time I was consulted by a patient that had a severe and rapidly progressive condition. In retrospect it is not uncommon to be treating a patient where the condition they have has passed a point where a full recovery is possible and this I consider was quite regretfully, true in this patient's case.

From previous conference work I had been shown a form of examination to test for single point genetic mutations.

This means in basic terms one "base" in the gene code has been substituted for another. Our gene code is made of bases denoted with the letters G, C, T, A which stand for (roughly!) Guanidine, Cytosine, Thymidine, and Adenine.

And so a single point mutation may have for example a G replaced by an A and thus the enzyme made from a copy of that mutated gene may thus work improperly and so eventually an "illness" would develop.

These single point mutations can affect genes which are required for the vitamins that we obtain from food to be converted into active forms called, coenzymes. These coenzymes are very important in that they are needed to make our enzymes work properly so as to run a healthy body or a healthy metabolism. Enzymes quite literally "run" our biochemistry.

If we have a very good genetic makeup, i.e. healthy genes we are more likely of course to feel well. A common illness for example, a viral infection, the virus "injects" it's genetic material into our cells, our own cells then "read" the viral DNA or RNA and thus new viruses are manufactured.

It is common that with a viral infection we feel unwell as a result of the virus producing material that upsets or blocks or poisons our normal functions. As an aside from my own clinical experience, a viral infection often has a characteristic of the sudden onset of substantial pain. If our immune system works well the virus is destroyed. If we are not running perfectly well I consider that our immune system may leave the job of destroying and or "eating up" the virus incomplete. That is we could be left with cells in our bodies that contain remnant parts or segments of the original viral DNA or RNA.

What I began to see in patients was the following. If I tested a patient against say fifty types of infection, generally they might demonstrate a response or reaction to two or three that I may consider as pernicious or low grade infections (chapter 6). If the testing performed was biased toward genetic material, DNA and or RNA, often then whereas there had been two or three responses in testing for an infection as a complete entity, I would then see five times that number of responses i.e. ten to fifteen. Hence I began to lean toward the idea that an entire microbial infection or its complete genetic compliment was not present yet segments of its genetic material remained and as such a causative factor with respect to illness.

If only a part or parts of the viral DNA were left behind there would not be whole new viruses being made in our cells, yet parts of the virus could be made. A segment of "infectious" DNA left behind could be "read" so that our cells could therefore make toxic material as an ongoing function. Thus to coin a term we could then have a cell which could be considered to be " AUTOTOXIC" or self-poisoning.

For many years in practice I had used quite a variety of treatment approaches. Having more "tools", one has a greater likelihood of finding tools which are most likely to suit the patient best. The use of herbal medicines, homeopathic medicines, treatment of the spine, acupuncture meridians, manually moving glands and organs, use of vitamins and coenzymes, minerals, massage and so on all worked well. Yet in approaching the theory of AUTOTOXCITY and treating that apparent "state" as best as I could see, this has enabled me to make a leap as such so that what I had previously used to treat a patient to "drive" a healthier metabolism or to detoxify a patient was either no longer required or of much less importance.

For example in years passed I would often supplement a patient with a vitamin or mineral and yet in treating what would appear to be an "AUTOXICITY", that supplemental requirement has all but disappeared!

Similarly I may have used say dandelion herb for example to detoxify a patient's liver and again now, my need to do this or repeat that process has diminished dramatically.

By way of analogy it is as if as a motor mechanic I have tried to make the car run much better and yet the hand brake has been pulled on a bit. Try and drive a car with the brake on and it doesn't go so well. Yet treatment with a view to removing what could appear to be DNA or RNA that is not ours or non self from infectious processes has so to speak taken the brakes off, made working with a patient easier and more successful!

My initial bias in treating what would appear to be retained or remnant nucleic acids (DNA, RNA) from microbial infections was to see if the use of common foods as "medicine" would be effective.

Importantly what I have found to be useful in treating the above may well be specific to the climate in which my patients live and how that genetic makeup functions within that climate. I work in a region where the weather pattern would be considered temperate, yet the majority of my patients would be primarily of British or northern European origin.

That is I am working predominantly with people who would come from a lineage more suited to a colder climate. As such what I have found to be effective within my own practice may or may not be as applicable or as effective across the genetic variance of other nationalities or race. I do though tend to err toward thinking that my approach could well be effective, for example treating someone of Mediterranean origins, living in a cold climate. That is though, of course only something that could be seen over time in treating large numbers of patients of various racial origins.

Furthermore even with a patient who would appear to have a significant level of "remnant microbial nucleic acids" I would not always treat that directly. That is in some patients if I had them temporarily include or eliminate a particular food, treat an infection, reduce their exposure to sources of infection or use a dietary roughage for example there would be what would appear to be an improvement in their apparent "genetic function" or a reduction in volume of "non self" genes, that is, a similar positive effect or result via different means.

What I have found to be useful in specifically aiming at "non self" DNA or RNA has been the following:

➢ Apricot or apricot kernel oil.

➢ Brazil nuts, possibly due to containing high levels of selenium cysteine.

➢ Raw oats or oat bran, possibly due to significant levels of the amino acid, lysine.

➢ Indian tonic water, effective agent possibly quinine.

➢ Coenzyme Q10 (ubiquinone)

The above seven foods or nutrients have for the most part been used one at a time or in isolation rather than in combination. My thinking is that each one of the above may have a separate function or specific action or is very likely to. Also that in using any one of the above there can be a multiplicity of effects, for example the selenium cysteine in brazil nuts may raise the levels of T3 (one of the thyroid hormones) .

Brazil nuts may provide oils which could improve cell membrane function, especially nervous system function. Oats or oat bran can be useful as a roughage to assist in removal of waste or toxic fats or unwanted steroid hormones or variants of steroid hormones. Coenzyme Q10 will often raise energy production within the body, though in general only where a deficiency of that molecule exists.

The adage that "food is the best medicine" it often seemed to me that food in itself would not be a powerful enough and yet with experience I believe it can be a very potent form of medicine. Consistent with this I have found that utilising small doses can be very effective for example often to "prescribe" no more than one Brazil nut a day for say seven days. Using a specific food as a medicinal intervention, especially a non staple food if used in

24

concert with other modalities, one does not often require a long term usage or large amounts. Occasionally I will find some problem with a patient in that they have had a quite tangible success by taking a particular food as a medicine and then they have "overdosed" by either eating too much or for too long.

In addition to using a food or foods to treat a particular complaint I almost invariably use physical means, for example, addressing the spine or skeletal muscles, lymphatic tissue, loosening facial restrictions affecting glands or organs, treatment of acupuncture meridian points and so forth. Use of physical or manual interventions does I feel reduce the requirement for larger intakes of some nutritional elements and I believe does work in a synergistic fashion.

Not only have the doses used been small, as above, in general they are not ongoing. By way of analogy, like filling the radiator in your motor vehicle with coolant, often once the required amount is there, you're done.

To point out the obvious, a patient would not be advised to take a food for which they have or have had an allergy or sensitivity to or suspicion of such. Of course, by example one would not have a patient eat Brazil nuts if there was a history of any adverse reaction to nuts.

A patient who alters their diet to attempt an improvement in their health is wise to do so only under professional guidance and here I am repeating myself to provide emphasis of the importance of this. Someone who is serious with regard to their health care is best advised to discuss potential changes with their practitioner. To exercise caution and assist that practitioner by being open and informative, this increases ones likelihood of success.

The effect of my use of the above foods has appeared as I have said to reduce need for detoxification, the use of vitamins and minerals, also to reduce the apparent load of what I would call pernicious infection.

In general terms, using food as a means to alter abnormal function, that is ill health, it has made the treatment of patients quicker, easier, more successful and more lasting. For me as a practitioner that is a happy thing and so as well for the patient. Once more, again seek advice first!

IS IT FAT?

Someone can be overweight or oversize not just from an excess of unwanted fat!

An overweight condition can be as a result of the following excesses, or in some cases paradoxically, deficiencies.

- ➢ Fats
- ➢ Oils
- ➢ Starches
- ➢ Fluid
- ➢ Gelatinous material
- ➢ Infectious material
- ➢ Waste protein
- ➢ Androgens
- ➢ Female hormones

I believe that many people would struggle with achieving a satisfactory and lasting weight loss in part due to approaches that are only or primarily aimed at losing fat.

A good place to begin is as always taking a detailed history of the patient's health. Identifying what as above is contributing to an overweight condition, that is what are the causative agents, is essential to providing effective treatment.

With respect to fats and oils being retained in excess, the causes of this as with most conditions can be both multiple and various.

With reference to chapter 5, (Roughage) I have seen dramatic successes utilising a roughage to "clean" the bile and so as to in a sense unblock that gall bladder / large intestine passage exit for unwanted fatty acids.

Five years ago a fellow consulted me with regard to a low back condition. It is not uncommon that gut dysfunction or more so, large intestine trouble can contribute to low back pain. The patient demonstrated what was consistent with a parasitic bowel infection. Some people are somewhat horrified at the idea of having a parasite infection, though they do exist and in my clinical experience, they are quite common infections.

The patient was prescribed an anti parasitic medication which was very effective not only in helping relieve his back pain but also in dramatically lowering his weight.

A weight loss of something in the vicinity of seven kilograms over a four week period, which I suppose is somewhat spectacular. I consider that a significant volume of that weight loss may well have been quite literally infectious material. This man reported that the volume of material he had been passing as 'stool' was enormous over the period of that treatment.

Importantly here the following idea may well have validity. If it is that pernicious or low grade infections are common it may be that these infections alter our biochemistry so as to "fatten" us up. Hence the infection has more material upon which to live and I suppose more space in which to reside. Not the most pleasant idea to consider. Yet in real terms if we look at life on this planet, living things both eat and are eaten. As the French expression, c'est la vie, c'est la guerre, in life without sufficient defence, someone or something may opportune to take from us. Or again maybe in not so pleasant terms, "we are all food for worms". It is a worthy consideration to avoid that while we are still alive !

What is a basic standpoint is the consideration that eating too much of a particular food or type of food is likely to upset our biochemistry yet also that if it is in excess we may just store it in the body and or provide "food" for an insidious infection!

This accumulation of "weight" may occur with fats, oil "starchy" food, protein, even water if too much is consumed. With respect to drinking water, I like the Chinese medical point of view that our urine is best a pale beer colour, too much water and the urine is clear, too little and it becomes dark. This is though a general consideration, patients under supervision for a specific condition or conditions would essentially be required to follow their practitioner's advice.

Occasionally I will hear women refer to their parts of excess size not as fat but as "jelly". If we were all perfectly well, then material such as glucosamine sulphate (water absorbent "padding" in our joints i.e. cartilage) would only be deposited where our bodies design dictates. In a patient with some level of abnormal function I consider that they may produce a "gelatinous like" material in their soft tissues from excesses and or poor handling of amino acids from protein and "sugars" or carbohydrates. The deposition of a gelatinous like material in the soft tissues thus contributing to that person's excess weight and relative appearance of being "fat".

As such in some cases, a patient attempting to lose weight may have more success via changing their protein, sugar or carbohydrate intake rather than simply lowering their consumption of fats. A dysfunctional metabolism may "think" "alright we have too much of a particular amino acid (from the excess of a particular food) we'll combine it with say glucose and make a jelly".

By way of example, I recently noticed that a colleague of mine had quite dramatically lost weight. She related to me that she had since her teenage years on almost a daily basis eaten a handful of various nuts as part of her diet. She attributed the loss of weight which was roughly a loss of five kilograms over something like a three or four month period to having stopped that consumption of nuts. That is one very simple change in a dietary habit resulting in a satisfactory loss of weight. It would be easy to say that the weight loss was from a reduced consumption of fats and oils contained within the nuts though it may have also been in part due to the change in her consumption of various proteins. And as with the above paragraph she may have had a loss of weight in part due to a loss of gelatinous material. A further consideration is that as nuts in general terms are "seeds" she may well have acquired an excess of nucleic acids or components of such or an adverse bias within her levels of purines and pyrimidine's.

These purines and pyrimidine's being "building blocks" of DNA and RNA. As such I consider that it is possible to adversely affect our production and repair of our own genes via inappropriate dietary choices. By way of analogy, a difficulty of achieving a specified building design due to an imbalance of bricks versus mortar.

Furthermore I consider that we may retain an excess of some fats in an attempt to have our biochemistry convert those fats into a type or types of fats that we do require and yet fail to do so. If we are unable to perform this function it is I believe possible to supplement a required fat or oil with a patient and thus achieve a loss in weight. Often though, I find there is a greater likelihood of success by temporarily removing one type of fat or oil and including one that is required.

One phenomenon I have seen is an apparent relationship between the following; parasite infections, calcium, fluoride (see chapter 7.) and male hormones, "androgens", (testosterone for example).

A patient of mine (female, a note, the majority of my patients are women) had complained of a history, of having for many years, morning diarrhoea. Upon examination I believe her complaint was due to a longstanding parasite infestation. She responded very well to simply using Indian tonic water (contains quinine which can be used as an anti parasitic medication). What struck me was that between that initial visit and the follow up, her appearance had changed dramatically.

She quite literally seemed to have lost such "bulk" that there was the appearance of her being less "wide" by a few centimetres. If there is a validity to the above association i.e. androgens and parasite infections, it would seem that her androgen levels had as a result of the treatment, lowered, hence a lesser appearance of a "masculine" bulk.

As above, an additional link or apparent link with respect to altering fluoride levels in a patient, often the resultant response would be a lesser propensity for a patient to sustain low grade infections, also a lesser need for dietary roughage and a more feminine or "prettier" facial appearance in my female patients.

Again as with any medicinal or dietary alteration it is wise to seek professional advice. It is not that one would think for example "maybe tonic water would be good for me" and then take it as an "experiment". Be careful, if you are serious about your health care do so in working with a qualified practitioner !

I have seen some patients apply some simple or "generic" approaches as a means to lose weight as follows. For example, within a program, taking longer periods of exercise of over forty minutes so that the duration of that exercise may be sixty to seventy minutes can increase the amount of fat used for energy production. That is in general we tend to "burn up" sugars first then switch more toward using up and breaking down fats by increasing the length of an exercise session. Again the wisdom here, seek advice, a professional trainer and or medical approval for an exercise program! Combining aerobic and anaerobic i.e. including weights to build muscle can also be helpful with a view to weight loss.

Most certainly chewing very thoroughly can help to achieve a loss of excess weight by reducing the amount of food required and making digestion and absorption easier. I recall hearing this suggestion and applying that eating dinner one night. If I chewed my food until I was only swallowing fluid it was a slow process, probably half an hour. Yet I was only able to eat a third of what was usual. Not that I had to lose weight though I felt it was sufficient for me to have eaten so little. That is in chewing thoroughly it maybe a simple way for some to take in sufficient nutrition even though they would eat a lesser amount and therefore lose weight as a result.

In the late eighties I consulted a naturopath who recommended avoiding the combination of protein with carbohydrate. That is for example if one ate fish not to include a starch, for example, potato, peas, pumpkin, rice. Part of the idea here is that the digestion of protein is primarily a stomach function, carbohydrate more of an exocrine pancreas, small intestine function. Including a starch with a protein tends to raise the propensity for the carbohydrate to absorb stomach digestive fluids and so limit digestion somewhat.

Occasionally with the above a patient may lose weight quickly and easily using one approach though usually a combination of approaches is required.

ROUGHAGE

Our bodies contain billions of cells. If you imagine these cells are like tiny bubbles containing our metabolic or biochemical "machinery". Within the outer cell "walls" we have another " little cell" or nucleus containing our chromosomes, i.e. our DNA, our genes. Within our cytoplasm or in lay terms, between our outer cell wall and the nucleus we have little organelles, for example our mitochondria which are the major site of energy production within the body.

These cell walls or membranes are made predominantly from "fatty acids" or fats and oils. A fatty acid is a chain of carbon atoms with hydrogen atoms attached and at one end of that chain is an "acid" group or in a language of chemistry a COOH group. The "fatty" part i.e. the carbon chain with hydrogen atoms attached is hydrophobic (not liking water). The "acid" group is hydrophilic or water loving.

So from the above our cell membranes are a double layer of fats and oils with the "fatty ends" together on the inside of the layer and the hydrophilic ends on the outside surface.

These fatty membranes are semipermeable, that is they selectively allow the passage in or out of various molecules, "atoms", ions so as to allow a flow of "electrical charge" and thus enable transmission of nerve "signals".

Our bodies are a self-healing self-cleaning or detoxifying and self-renewing. Remove what is blocking or poisoning our natural functions and provide what we need to function normally, provide some rest and we tend toward healing, repair, or a renewing that is a process toward health. I like to think the best part of health is happiness. If we feel well, life is easier.

Our fats and oils are constantly being renewed or replaced. It is said that in a seven year period we have a "new body" hence "the seven year itch". These fats and oils are removed from our cell walls when "old" or "oxidised" then transported on carriers, dissolved in the bile in our liver/gall bladder. When we eat a meal, the liver/gall bladder bile is squeezed into our intestines where it "sticks" to roughage in our food. Through the small then large intestine the fats pass out in our stool.

The point here is that roughage can be used as a cleaning or clearing agent to assist in the emptying of unwanted or old fats and oils from our bile, from our bodies. Roughage therefore is an essential element within our diet.

Where a patient is deficient in roughage or other essential nutrition or has a "mild" infection that may upset our normal functions, we can then reabsorb fats back up into our liver / gall bladder rather than emptying them out. This is of course not an uncommon means by which people can become " FAT " !

Failure to remove unwanted fats or oils can prevent us from having "space" in the bile to absorb new healthy fats. If our cell walls become clogged with old fats and deficient in those fats we need, then our cells don't work so well, especially so within our nervous system !

In some cases a patient may lose a great deal of weight by using roughage to assist in the removal of unwanted fat. Of course the use of roughage is not a requirement in all cases.

Occasionally I have seen a spectacular loss of weight in patients simply with the use of a roughage as a "medicine" or for example a satisfactory reduction with the experience of "hot flushes". In part, a roughage can be used detoxify fat soluble waste within the liver and so lower its metabolic "heat". Also as processed or used oestrogens or progesterone pass out in the stool a patient can rid themselves of those and other unwanted steroid hormones that can contribute to trouble with menstruation.

As our fatty cell membranes hold cell "receptors" which receive instructive "signals", our bodies communication can improve or the cell can better know what to do if it is that we have healthy or appropriate levels of specific fats and oils within those membranes or cell walls. Also, the fatty cell membranes contain or hold "ports" or "gates" so we may with using a roughage, enable a cell to take in more easily what it needs and pass out waste material more effectively so as to achieve a more functional level of signalling within the body.

Our brain, our nervous system is made of cells, as like others, with fatty membranes. Poor fat content within our nerves can contribute to mental and emotional upset! A simple example to provide here was the treatment of young female patient.

She complained not so much of depression, more of feeling unwell mentally or despondent or feeling unpleasant in her mind. A major part of the treatment was having her take a roughage over a three week period. Within seven days she reported to be feeling much better. After three weeks and only two clinical visits she was in my estimation, well enough and quite apparently, much happier. Doing the work that quickly and easily with such a good response is a very gratifying thing, well I think for me and the patient.

One further example, one that I would consider to have been quite spectacular is the following. Six years ago a woman in her mid fifties consulted me with a number of complaints. The one pertaining to this example was that she suffered a somewhat debilitating arthritic condition in her knee's. The most significant nutritional approach that she followed was to eat, to chew thoroughly and swallow approximately one dessertspoon of oat bran on a daily basis for one week. The severity of her arthritis was such that she had for a few years been unable to dance for more than only very short periods, maybe a song or two. Dancing was I think one of her favourite recreations and as such she was somewhat distressed with this lack of capacity. To my surprise at her second consultation she related to me that on the previous evening she had been able to dance for over an hour and a half without undue distress.

It would not at all be that every case of arthritis would respond so well or so quickly yet that was the response in her case. I suppose an understatement to say that was a good result!

Why the above effect or result? The human body is extraordinarily complex and so it would be difficult to guess as to exactly what biochemical changes where responsible for the patient's improvement though the following may be a useful "model" to consider. If it was that her bile was in a rough language "full of old fats and oils" and therefore much less able to uptake new or healthy fats and oils then she may have suffered significantly from a deficiency of requisite oils within her joints. The synovial fluid which provides lubrication within a joint does require a level of oils. And so as a theoretical perspective it may be that the oat bran "cleared" her bile to an extent that enabled the uptake of sufficient oils so as to "relubricate" her knee's and thus provide a welcome functional change.

What I have used as a roughage for patients to take is the following:

> Raw or cooked oats (usually raw)
> Oat bran
> Desiccated coconut
> Rice bran
> Wheat bran

Importantly, even though a patient may have an excess retention of fats, I will not always use a roughage as a means to help remove those fats. Again as with treating "remnant microbial" genetic material, usually only one agent is used and for a limited time often not greater than two weeks. As with all suggestions for a patient with respect to using a food substance, one will not use a food where there is a history of or suspicion of the food contributing to a sensitivity or causing an allergic reaction i.e. caution is paramount.

There is a tendency with patients if a particular food has worked well, i.e. brought about a good result, for them to want to use it in an ongoing fashion. Often the use of one food once the job is done it is best to stop. Just as one would fill their petrol tank once it's full, there is no need to continue until there is a further need.

The use of a roughage with patients is along similar lines to much of what is within the content of this book, it is something that is inexpensive, easy to use and often very effective !

PERNICIOUS INFECTION

Within the process of persistently looking for the cause and more often, the causes of a patient's condition, the commonness of very low grade infection has become to me quite evident.

An infection of a serious nature would essentially require medical attention. That could include in some cases or a cold, a flu, abscess or gastric infection for example. A pernicious infection would be considered as one much less acute less obvious than the above or of a lesser severity. Pernicious may be described as harmful in a gradual or subtle way, or insidious. By way of an analogy, a cold or flu or infection requiring immediate medical attention could be seen as running the taps to fill a bath with water. A pernicious infection could be seen as a dripping tap, an ongoing agent that in time may contribute significantly to illness, fatigue, biochemical abnormality. Also one that may not be evident with the use of some laboratory tests. Most people are aware of having a cold or flu or gastric upset and they would often attribute those conditions and symptoms to an infection. Often in the common language it would be said they have a virus, though I consider from experience they may just as likely be suffering a bacterial, fungal or parasite infection or combinations of these agents. A pernicious, or pernicious infections are very commonly what I would find as causative or contributing factors to many human ailments, for example back pain, headache, neck pain, osteoporosis, arthritis, fatigue, postural distortions, mental / emotional conditions. Some of the most profound changes or improvements that I have seen in many long term or chronic conditions have been via reducing a patients exposure to infectious material and eliminating or reducing that excess infectious load within their body !

Reducing what I believe is an excess of infectious processes can free a patient's biochemistry so that there is a bias more toward energy for activity, detoxification healing and repair. By way of analogy one could imagine that a patient with a chronic and excess infectious load as would a country be at war and as such sustain an ongoing drain upon their resources.

The home environment is I think so very important, for example a patient who sleeps on an old mattress infected with "microfauna" may be bitten frequently with dust mites, insects of various types. If it is that we can acquire malaria (a parasitic infection) from a mosquito bite, then I believe that we can acquire infections from agents within our mattress, pillows, carpet, pets, poorly serviced air-conditioning.

Over the years I have often recommended a patient replace an old mattress. Not uncommonly they would remark that the new mattress did not feel so different in its firmness yet they may have felt their back pain for example much reduced or that they had slept better and felt more refreshed in the morning.

An old mattress can accumulate a large volume of perspiration, oils from our bodies, dust, dead skin, which can be a source of food for what would live within a mattress or pillow. Using a mattress protector that can be thoroughly cleaned is a good idea. I would suggest that once a mattress is seven to eight years old, it has done it's time. For pillows, every one to two years is a reasonable replacement time frame.

Carpet if very old is better either replaced or removed so as to have bare wood or tiles, and the use of rugs that can be are more easily aired or cleaned.

It is easy for air-conditioning systems to acquire populations of infectious matter, especially so with recycling evaporative units. Where possible, fans and open windows are a far healthier option. Regular servicing, cleaning and replacement of filters with air conditioners with the use of professional contractors, is I consider a very important exercise. Reverse cycle units may be in general a better option than the evaporative units, in that they have a lesser propensity to introduce moisture into a home or office which would facilitate the growth of mould or fungus for example which can be extremely toxic. I would like to emphasise though many people would not consider air conditioning as a danger to their health I do believe they can be extremely dangerous!

With regard to jet lag, I do believe that part of the effects that someone may experience, fatigue at least is as result of having been exposed to a relatively high concentration of airborne infectious material. As a means to counteract the above, I have had patient's report that they had had a lesser experience of what they would describe as jet lag by employing the following. One, attempting to counter the respiration of airborne infections by simply using an intranasal application of proprietary Vicks Vaporub. Secondly as a means to counter an acquired infection or infections by consuming small amounts of Indian Tonic Water and with regard to "small amounts" only one or two small bottles. Patients that I have that fly very regularly are tested or examined so that I can be more specific and varied to their requirements at least in part here that the ongoing use of one type of treatment rarely sustains a successful result without employing some variation. In other words one approach may work well for a time and then come to a point where its effectiveness is either lost or would begin to become detrimental.

The smoking of cigarettes or cigars is considered to be a significant health hazard and yet I believe that what is contained within the air from some air conditioning units could be far worse, as follows. Firstly some fungal toxins for example are of an extreme level of toxicity. With cigarette smoke there is a toxicity, yet with the use of an air conditioner we can quite literally be inhaling live infectious microorganisms. In addition whereas with a cigarette the inhalation is usually oral, with a "septic" air conditioning system there is a nasal intake. Please note I am not here suggesting someone would take up smoking. This "septic air" introduces the possibility of infectious microorganisms entering and progressing into our olfactory and facial nerves. I consider that from such infection's there exists the potential for an encephalitis to develop, i.e. an infection within the brain.

A pernicious or subclinical encephalitis is within my clinical experience not so uncommon. Of course such an infection is something which can be extremely dangerous. Where possible it is I think a far safer alternative to be using ceiling or exhaust fans and open windows in preference to air conditioners. As above if you are to use an air conditioning system make sure it is cleaned and serviced thoroughly and regularly. With some units it is recommended that they be serviced biannually though I would be more inclined to make that three or four times a year.

Pets in the home can be a tremendous source of pleasure yet if they carry infectious material this can be a contributing factor with respect to a patient's having an ongoing low grade infection.

The best source of advice in this regard of course would be your veterinary surgeon. Proper care of your pet is not only good for them but also for those whom they live with.

A clean house or work place is not so much a cure in itself, although it is likely to make an improvement in ones health and so as to enable it to be easier for your practitioner to care for you. By way of example, five years ago, I had a patient with an " eczema-like", skin condition. It was for her a source of pain, irritation, fatigue and insomnia. Before taking on what I had prescribed for her she moved to a new apartment, had a new mattress, pillows and linen. She remarked that the skin condition had disappeared within a few days. It is a happy thing for a practitioner and certainly the patient, to have such a result via such simple means.

Very few things in life are always. It is not to say that a low grade infection is present in all conditions yet I consider it is very common.

With the accumulation of years it is common to see on x-ray, degeneration of the spine. I used to think this was simply some process of aging or mechanical damage from heavy manual labour, which of course it can be. Yet in some cases where the discs of the lumbar spine degenerate and flatten, there can be I believe the presence of a slow or "quiet" infectious process gradually eating the fibrous or connective tissue which makes up the disc. Also that a similar process can occur within our bones. Not only can the patient thus experience pain due to mechanical distortion of a degenerating disc or vertebra, yet also suffer pain from toxic material produced or waste released from the residing infectious microorganisms.

Furthermore within the cycle of an infection or infections, the bodies repair or healing processes to regenerate tissues can be a source of pain in itself.

Any tissue or body part can be availed to an infection, be that a joint, bone, organ or gland, the nervous system, brain for example, the skin or gut.

I recall the first statement spoken by my second year university physiology lecturer was "that there are more nerve cells in the gut than there are in the brain". And so a gut, stomach, small or large intestine or less specifically, liver, gall bladder, spleen or pancreatic infection may well have an adverse and profound effect upon our nervous system. Not dissimilarly within the skin (the largest organ of the body), a chronic low grade infectious process can provide significant neural or nervous system irritation.

As "digested" food is absorbed from our gut through the gut walls, collected within the blood and transported in the portal vein to the liver, as such a chromic gut infection can be a major source not only of infection but also toxicity within the liver and gall bladder.

A low grade gut infection can easily cause indigestion, be a major contributing factor to experiencing food sensitivities, a dysfunctional nervous system, mental emotional trouble, fatigue, body odour, skin conditions for example.

Such low grade infection is more likely to be within the province of naturopathic medicine or other so called alternative medicines. Importantly though, I believe the choice of what type of practitioner or practitioners a patient is to see must be those in which the patient has faith. My bias is toward as would be called alternative medicine, though I have myself been able to find help with conventional medical practitioners and pharmaceutical medicines. Seeing a practitioner with whom you are happy and their chosen modality is very important.

As above, a naturopath, a doctor of Chinese or ayuvedic medicine for example may well be more adept or conscious of treating a low grade or pernicious infections as such. Often conventional naturopathy will treat the gut as a standard part of their approach, usually by prescribing oral medicines I have heard it said that if you "fix the gut" then you will be seventy per cent of the way there. I am aware though of the powerful effect that can be achieved by using external treatments. In my view using only oral medicines may well not be entirely effective to treat minor infections within the skin, muscle, ligamentous tissues or bone. A referral to a qualified AROMATHERAPIST may be in such cases a very good option.

Using herbal medicines orally is one way to impart a useful herbal remedy into the body. Using oils as carriers and applied to the skin can be very effective in that the then medicine surrounds the body. Also, a qualified aromatherapist may well be able to prescribe oils to use in the home as part of a medicinal approach and or to improve the hygiene within the home environment. HOMEPATHIC medicine is also a powerful and viable approach at least in part in that it is safe, inexpensive and can be diffuse in effect.

Some simple examples here may provide illustration. Ten years ago a patient consulted me within a complaint of low back pain. As an aside, apart from a low thoracic manual adjustment the recurrence of the fellow's pain was largely eliminated by having him avoid milk for a time and from then only taking small amounts. That is, the intolerance to milk had an effect that was substantial enough within his gut so as to cause sufficient irritation within his nervous system to reflect in muscle imbalances and thus back pain.

What more took my interest though, within this fellow's right hand was a condition of DUPUYTRENS CONTRACTURE. The patient had had previously, one surgical intervention which was somewhat successful yet after eighteen months the contracture had returned to almost it's original severity. The man's surgeon had given him the option of a second operation yet pointed out that the outcome may in time be similar to that of the first attempt.

Testing of this right hand displayed indications of a FUNGAL infection. What appeared to negate this fungus was simply, tea tree oil. Three or four applications of tea tree oil were used upon the right hand and arm over a period approximately two weeks.

Within a three week period the contracture had all but disappeared. Remaining was some shortening of tissues along the previous surgical scars though for the most part the functioning of his hand had become near normal. Upon seeing the fellow eighteen months later to consult regarding a different complaint, his right hand was still quite satisfactory.

Please note, this is not at all to say that a dupuytrens contracture is always caused by a fungal infection, the causes are as with most condition likely to be various. Also even though the patient responded well to topical use of the tea tree oil, again this is not to say that approach would be effective either with all fungal infections or all cases of dupuytrens contracture.

Essentially my approach was to attempt to identify a causative agent and then an application which would effectively treat that condition. Conversely in many cases rather than utilising an agent to kill an infection it can be effective to eliminate a food or foods that would seem to be "feeding" that infection, then rely upon the patient's own immune system to deal with the infection. Also of course as above, to attempt to identify any environmental source of that infection or similar infections so as to reduce the likelihood of persistence or recurrence.

There is a large volume of nerves within the skin! Of Chinese medical philosophy the lungs are the organs of emotion, the lungs govern the skin and hair. Thus not only can an external treatment such as the use of an aromatherapy oil or mix of oils benefit various glands or organs but then also have a direct effect upon the nervous system within the skin. Similarly' using an oil burner to "vaporise" a medicinal oil, there is here an exposure to the skin and an entry into the body via respiration within the lungs.

Varying or being specific in choosing the region of entry or application of a medicine i.e. via oral means to gut, topically to the skin or via respiration with an "oil burner" for example can be of enormous benefit in addressing a given health condition quickly and effectively.

In simple terms a hygienic home and work environment, careful consideration of what food is consumed, working with a qualified practitioner can enable a patient to lower their infectious load to a point where their own immune system is then able to deal effectively with the "normal" exposure within those environments. A patient that is not overwhelmed by or subject to an excessive infectious "load" is far more likely to experience a better level of health, a better sense of wellbeing !

FLUORIDE

Altering the intake of fluoride in a patient can in my experience have a very powerful and positive effect upon that patients health. I would emphasise this point as it does seem to be a somewhat obscure idea though now in my clinical practice it is an essential consideration. It would appear that the use of fluoride especially within toothpaste has had a beneficial effect upon the health and strength of our teeth. I would see or hear three different views with respect to the use of fluoride, one that is a good thing, two that it is toxic or harmful, and three, no view at all or at least no consideration the importance of its use.

I believe that the fluoride levels within our bodies not only affect the amount of calcium within our teeth but also the relative levels that exist between our bones and our "soft tissues". Soft tissues meaning for example our muscles and ligaments. Also that fluoride levels can affect the relative levels of both calcium and magnesium within our nervous system, our glands and organs.

The balance and distribution of calcium and magnesium within our body is very important, exceptionally so! The following points may provide some understanding here.

> Magnesium is very much required to attach to many of the enzymes that we make in the body. These enzymes are made from the expression of our genetic code and quite literally "run" our metabolism, our biochemistry.

> Magnesium is very important with regard to both energy production in the body and for our ability to be able to relax muscles or switch muscles off.

> Calcium is both an on switch in the brain and as such an on switch in our muscles. An excess load of calcium can very well contribute to fatigue within both our nervous system and our muscles, the experience of cramps or "restless" legs for example.

> Both calcium and magnesium are required for healthy bones.

> Calcium is required for our use of glycogen and so therefore has an influence upon our sugar metabolism.

➢ An excess level of calcium intake can somewhat alkalinise the stomach. The stomach requires sufficient acidity so as to "digest" and absorb minerals. Thus paradoxically to much ingestion of calcium may contribute to a poorer digestive capacity, lower absorptive function and thus lead to a weakening of our bones

Most people dose their mouths with fluoride toothpaste three or four times a day. Some would on a regular or occasional basis receive a fluoride treatment from their dentist and of course many would acquire fluoride from tap water. Fluoride is an important element within our immune system.

We use what are called reactive oxygen species as a means to "kill" infections in our bodies. Fluoride is required to make one of these essential reactive oxygen "chemicals"

Just as a level of deficiency of a particular nutrient within the body can lead to ill health, similarly an excess level can also be a cause of trouble. It is very much my experience in practice that the majority of my patients have had adverse effects from excess levels of fluoride and have responded very well not to the cessation or elimination of fluoride but to a reduction in their use or exposure to that element. The above is somewhat an understatement in that not only have some of the responses in patients been quite substantial, yet I feel in many cases without "normalising" a patients fluoride levels, it is often far more difficult to either sustain or achieve satisfactorily further improvements in levels of health or experience of unwanted symptoms.

By way of analogy, if the injection system of the motor in our car "floods" a cylinder with an excess of fuel there can there not only be a waste of fuel, a build up of unwanted deposits yet also a reduction in power. Similarly it would appear from my experience that excess levels of fluoride can lead to an excess of calcium in soft tissues, brain, glands, organs and so contribute to dysfunction and diminished health.

The opposite, a deficiency of fluoride can be a problem. As above some people consider that fluoride is bad and so that it should be avoided. It is common that in patients that I have seen that have for long periods of time used only a non fluoride toothpaste that they are as a result suffering a deficiency. I would more commonly see this in patients who have a bias toward "alternative" health care. On average it would appear that with patients, most seem to function somewhat better to the use of a non fluoride toothpaste on five or six days of a week and a standard fluoride toothpaste one to two days a week.

This is not a hard and fast rule as such, with some patients they appear to either need or tolerate well, the daily use of a common fluoride toothpaste. Those that have an aversion to common commercial pastes may respond well to the occasional use of a simple proprietary calcium fluoride "tissue salt", (calc fluor).

As an example, a single clinical experience, the following. I have for a number of years had as a patient a naturopath who had only made use of a non fluoride toothpaste for a considerable length of time. She is a most attractive girl as someone you might see in a fashion magazine, she presented on this occasion complaining predominantly of quite substantial fatigue, and by appearance, somewhat haggard.

The physical treatment that I employed differed very little with that from of previous visits though a degree of testing performed was consistent with her having a lower than "normal" level of fluoride. I suggested that either she would use a fluoride toothpaste for a week to raise her levels or to take a limited dosage of homeopathic calcium fluoride.

Upon the subsequent visit one week later, the change in her facial appearance was as if she looked five years younger. She did report that her sense of fatigue had all but passed. This is of course only one example and I do see a variety of other functional and symptomatic changes with the alteration of fluoride levels though it did impress me that there was such an apparent change in this girl with the alteration of only one simple variable.

To gain a better "picture" of responses with patients with respect to altering fluoride levels I would think it would take another three or four years in practice to do so. Yet one other response may seem apparent in that with a high local level of fluoride within the oral cavity there would appear not uncommonly to be raised levels of male hormones i.e. androgens. As such in some female patients that have exclusively used fluoride toothpaste, there would appear to be an excessive growth of hair across the upper lip. It is common in general terms having made an alteration to fluoride levels that over a period of time, the patients would tend to look younger and "carry" less weight.

Not only does it seem apparent in many cases that a patient may have an excess level of fluoride in their body, yet as it is that we only apply toothpaste in our mouths, I believe this can in addition lead to a greater and as such localised toxicity within the head and neck. As it is that our brain resides within our cranial vault, "our skull" and that I believe there exists the potential for excess levels of fluoride to raise calcium levels in neural tissue and as such therefore contribute to inappropriate and excess "firing" within our brain.

To have proper or healthy function in our nervous system it is important in that a nerve should only switch on when it is required to do so. If nerves do switch on inappropriately it is then an adverse function which can be a cause trouble. For example if we experience an excessive firing of nerves that produce noradrenalin, we may then experience the discomfort of anxiety. Excessively raised serotonin levels may contribute to a headache or migraine.

As an analogy, if one had the experience of their motor car suddenly "taking off" at a red light, this of course would not likely be a pleasant experience. Whatever can be done with a patient to prevent excessive firing of nerves will help prevent the experience of unwanted symptoms, especially fatigue and in addition reduce the rate at which our brain cells die !

It may seem to a patient that changing the toothpaste that they are using, be a relatively trivial exercise and yet as above in my experience that in doing so there can be very positive change in the patient's health and sense of wellbeing. Again importantly, with a patient who is under the supervision of a practitioner for any particular condition, it is very important that the practitioner is aware of and approves of any change that the patient may undertake. It is your health, that is to say, take care with it !

AN ANCESTRAL DIET

There are such a large number of theories with respect to what is best for us to eat either when we are well or when suffering an illness.

One particular idea or consideration which I have found very useful is to simply consider a patient's genetic heritage. Please note that this perspective would only be a part of what apply with respect to how I would advise one of my patients. If a patient has come from a long line of one particular race it would be expected that they would have a genetic make-up that has undergone a process of ''Darwinian" selection, to be more suited to the food that their ancestors ate and environment in which those ancestors lived.

One of the most common examples of the above that I'd see, would be in regard to the consumption of olive oil. I am not here at all being disparaging about olive oil yet it would appear that some people are very well suited to it and others are not.

Often in practice I would see what appears to be an adverse response to olive oil. Of course with some people it would very much contribute to their wellbeing.

It would appear to me that patients from Mediterranean origins or in part Mediterranean origins can do well using olive oil either for cooking or adding the oil unheated to their food. Yet patients of British, Nordic or northern European origins often respond very well in my experience to either limiting the use of olive oil or in some cases eliminating it from their diet.

The most common response I would see with a reduction in the use of a particular oil is a change in the patient's mood or mental emotional wellbeing (see chapter 12, mental emotional conditions).

In basic terms so much of our brain and nervous system is dependent upon its content and distribution of fats and oils. And so often, removing from the diet a fat or oils which are in excess and often then replacing that fat or oil with another can bring about a desired response.

Someone say of Scottish ancestry or Norwegian ancestry may well be better suited to eating animal or fish oils rather than say olive oil. They may also not be so well disposed to eating canola or sesame oil for example. This is not to say that in some instances these oils could be used for short periods of time as food or medicine.

Also the suitability of one food for someone say of northern Irish decent may be different for that person if they moved to another country, another climate. As such I will always use some form of testing to see if I can find some indication of what food is best suited at a particular time or at a particular state of health.

With the advent of refrigeration, what was that? nineteen twenties, it is now possible to eat in autumn or winter what our ancestors may only have been able to eat in summer or spring. What may be healthy to eat in summer may be not so or not at all beneficial in winter.

Again as with the genetic capacity of a particular race with many people being suited to particular food types or climate, we may feel better not eating the same things all year around. This from the simple perspective that our ancestors in general would have had to "cycle" the food that they ate as seasonally required.

As such, not only could it be that someone of Nordic origins be less suited to regularly eating coloured salad vegetables, they may be even less suited to do so in autumn or winter.

Some vegetables do contain enzymes that will switch on or "activate" vitamins in our bodies. If we have a "genetic line" which does not require so much of these enzymes then as with most dietary intake, too much of one food or type of good can cause trouble.

There is much information I suppose in "media health care" that would suggest broccoli is very good for you. This may be the case though some people in my experience do not tolerate broccoli so well. These patients may well have an ancestral history where their predecessors had never eaten it. And so there may be chemical constituents or compounds which they are unable to digest or process sufficiently, hence a propensity for something to contribute to abnormal function, to cause illness.

At least two elements to consider, in particular with broccoli, one a high level of salicylates and secondly high levels of chlorophyll.

Firstly high levels of salicylates in the diet may well not be in itself the cause of a "sensitivity" or gut sensitivity yet simply be an adverse response to an excess of that substance. Raised salicylates can elevate histamine levels. Excess histamine can present as redness, swelling, pain, irritation, "inflammation" as such. So in some cases a patient with a skin irritation or inflammation may respond well to either limiting or avoiding broccoli or other dark green leafy vegetables so as to lower or normalise their levels of salicylates and chlorophyll. Of course a patient may have been recommended to eat broccoli by a practitioner for other specific reasons and so again, first seek advice and follow what your practitioner has directed!

A vegetable high in chlorophyll may not be well suited in large amounts with a patient say of predominantly northern origins with pale skin living in a sunny climate.

Chlorophyll is a light sensitive molecule and of course of a green colour. Someone of pale complexion is more likely to have an adverse reaction to light impacting upon excess levels of chlorophyll within their body than someone with a relatively dark skin. Colour and light does affect our biochemistry! Eating too much of a food of one particular colour can upset a patients chemical or metabolic functions!

If a patient has a somewhat mixed genetic background, they may well be very lucky in being able to tolerate and improve their health with a wide range of foods.

I think maybe four factors have produced in society or a least what I have seen within my clinical experience, what for some patients have lead to an excess consumption of coloured fruit and salad vegetables.

Post Second World War, as foods that were rationed or unavailable were again on offer and may well have rebounded in consumption to excess levels. At least in Australia post war, the influx of Mediterranean market gardeners lead to the production of an abundance of very high quality fruit and vegetables. This bias though may well have less suited those of more northern origins.

There has been enormous scientific research into the value of quite a range of foods, though I pose the question… how much do you have? Some patients may do very well with small amounts of a good thing.

It is common to hear or to read that it is best to eat a "balanced" diet. My own experience was to have acquired a much greater sense of wellbeing, by altering my diet to consume food which in combination would be considered to be unbalanced. As such my health responded very well to an alteration so as to on only rare occasions i.e. maybe four or five times a year consume coloured or salad vegetables. For example I may only eat broccoli or red capsicum or asparagus as above, four or five times a year and any fruit two or three times a year. I am as far as I am aware predominantly of a northern European or Baltic lineage or genetic makeup and so in general terms I have largely reduced or eliminated food that would be more available or prevalent in a Mediterranean climate or Asian regions. As previously anyone with any medical condition and especially those already on a prescribed dietary regime would not proceed to alter their diet without further and specific advice from a medical or appropriately qualified practitioner !

The last twenty years has seen a proliferation of dietary books, magazine articles and especially television food or cooking programmes. What looks beautiful on a plate tends to be more of a Mediterranean or Asian cooking, of course not exclusively so. This may be the best food for people of those backgrounds or mixed ancestry and may be somewhat less so for people outside those "gene pools".

Simply put, consider what you eat, discuss with your practitioner what foods may be best suited to you and which ones may be best minimised or cycled, eaten seasonally or avoided.

JEWELLERY / METALS

The same theme, as with the majority of this book, to pursue the question, "what is it that may be having an adverse effect upon a patient which is then contributing to their illness or complaint"?

My training was primarily conventional and as with much of what I have written here, over time solutions have appeared which would seem unusual or unconventional, (this is probably somewhat an understatement!). Though some aspects of treatment or advice though seemingly out of the ordinary I believe what is most important is to pursue that which brings about not only a positive change in a patients function but also their symptomatic display, their sense of wellbeing. And so this chapter is along those lines, sometimes or I could say commonly, a spectacular improvement in a patient can be achieved by unusual means.

It is not within the scope of this book to discuss mercury toxicity or dental fillings in details though succinctly I would say in my experience patients with dental filling containing mercury do not do well. That comment would be very much an understatement!

There is much research on the subject of dental amalgam though I shall leave that and move on to the following.

If you were to see the best acupuncturist on the planet, it is very unlikely that he or she would leave an acupuncture needle in the body for a period of years or decades. Ears that are pierced, containing an earring or stud can behave as if treated with an acupuncture needle. Acupuncture can be a very powerful modality. Placing a needle into a meridian point or points can produce extraordinary improvements in a patient's health. Yet leaving a needle in a point for many years I believe can be very adverse. A similar theme here with respect to the use of certain foods, small amounts can be of great benefit, ongoing or large amounts may produce a great deal of trouble.

Of Chinese medical philosophy, the kidneys "govern the bones" and "govern" the ears. Kidney and bladder function or renal function is very much influenced by the neurotransmitter or "brain chemical" SEROTONIN. Too much serotonin and there is a tendency toward the experience of MIGRAINE HEADACHE. From a holographic perspective the ear may be seen as a baby upside down in the womb, the ear lobe as the head.

An internet search would show diagrams of acupuncture points within the ear. The lobe of the ear contains a cephalic point (head), a sensory, auditory and a "sneezing" point.

The insertion of needles into the pinna (external part) of the ear i.e. auricular acupuncture has been used for example to treat heroin addiction. If you can relieve an addiction of such voracity with acupuncture, then you could also increase the propensity for addiction in a similar way.

Not only can an earring or stud as it were, act like an acupuncture needle, it can produce a metal toxicity with the lobe and I have found that where the lobe is holed, there is a greater likelihood of localised infection.

I have not used the removal of earrings entirely as such in isolation and so with as always, other variables being present within the treatment of a patient it is difficult to quantify the effect of the removal of earrings so easily, though it is possible to see changes in simple neurological and manual muscle tests as a response following the removal of an earring or stud.

Two other common locations for studs are the eyebrow and the navel. Often an eyebrow stud will pass through or close to triple warmer 23 or triple heater 23. This can therefore affect thyroid and other endocrine or hormonal functions.

A navel stud will sit on or within the conception vessel acupuncture meridian and thus may affect DOPAMINE levels. It is not uncommon that a navel stud will affect low back pain and upset a patient's ability to flex or extend their body, that is, to be able to bend forward or backwards.

Three cases as examples, I believe that responded very well and significantly in my opinion from the cessation of the use of earrings, one firstly, a twenty nine year old woman with a prolonged history of classic migraine. Her migraines began at about age thirteen. She also had had her ears pierced in her early teens. She could not recall which came first, the migraine or the earring's, though I believe the ears being pierced may very likely have contributed to the onset of her condition. Within roughly two weeks of having removed the rings her symptoms had halved, within a month the migraines were gone.

Similarly a sixteen year old girl who had a diagnosed "panic disorder" and headache, demonstrated signs upon testing that were consistent with her earrings contributing to elevated levels of serotonin. Within three weeks she reported that she felt very much better to a point where I did not consider that she required further treatment.

A female patient whom I had treated over a number of years for a complaint of pelvic / sacroiliac pain and instability responded very well, simply in this case to abstaining from use of her earrings. The treatment approach at the time was along similar lines to what I had applied previously and so the only new variable was for the most part the removal of her earrings. She related to me that prior to disuse, her pelvis had not been stable enough to sustain running or jogging. Yet within two weeks she was able to run without having the previous discomfort.

Removal of earrings or studs is not a cure in itself for any particular condition yet I have found in many cases while the studs were in place, the successful resolution of a particular problem was not possible or the desired result unsatisfactory.

Some patients may tolerate their jewellery well enough. It is though common to see positive changes in simple neurological reflexes and manual muscle tests via the removal of particular items. Removal of individual or at times all rings, chains, studs, watches can be of great assistance in treating a patient. It is also a reasonably safe and easy thing to do.

As with earrings, a metal ring on a finger or toe or thumb can overtime impart a toxicity. Occasionally a patient will remark that having removed a ring there remains a black or black/green mark. This may seem to be trivial yet in treating a patient within limits it is often necessary to reduce aggravating factors as much as possible. Rare is it in my experience, that someone can make one change and suddenly acquire perfect health. Usually a patient requires removal of a combination or series of causative factors, provision of required nutrition and often especially a series or layers of treatment and changes.

If you looked at an internet search, it can be seen that acupuncture meridians run through the trunk, limbs, head and neck. I very much suspect that these meridian pathways within the skin and internally within the body may well be axonal or astrocyte like, i.e. neuronal or not dissimilar to nerve pathways.

As with the above paragraph, here is the potential for a piece of jewellery to be toxic i.e. to ''poison'' a particular acupuncture point or meridian pathway.

In addition, not only nerves within the skin and possibly with acupuncture meridians, if it is that they have a neuronal like behaviour they may well react to electrical currents, magnet fields or electromagnetic radiations or the presence of metals. As the flow of ions or potential difference set up via ions within and surrounding a nerve are tiny, it is plausible that they may easily be upset by what would appear to be some trivial influence for example, a metal ring or stud.

It is not uncommon within my practice to see a gross muscle weakness for example, a psoas muscle "strengthen" satisfactorily simply by removing the ring on a finger or toe ring or neck chain. The psoas major is a large muscle running at the front and either side of the lumbar spine. As such it is a primary stabiliser within the lumbar spine and pelvis. That is not to say that the removal of a ring would be all that would be required to have that muscle function properly. Yet in some cases the change in a muscle's response, strength and power can be quite startling.

Not dissimilarly I consider wrist watches can also be a source of aggravation. If you searched , "SENSORY HOMUNCULUS", it is evident from such diagrams that the sensory input to the brain from the upper limbs, especially hands and wrist, is large in comparison to many other parts or structures. As with the "dripping tap" theory in respect of low grade infections, I consider that long term, a wrist watch can confer a "plastic" change within the nervous system and so thus, the body, therefore to contribute to distortion, dysfunction.

Some patients do have a strong emotional or preferential attachment to a piece of jewellery. I do not like to be overly commanding in the giving of instructions to patients. Something of great sentimental value may be of a more overall positive value than that which may be of a physically detrimental effect. A patient may be happy enough to go "half way" and remove jewellery of an evening to sleep or use on only special occasions. Importantly, a patient may be somewhat overwhelmed by an illness or a particular condition. It is often little use to try to insist they do something that they feel unable to do. This applies not only to jewellery but changes in diet or habits or home environment and to the physical treatment of that patient. A predisposition to be gentle toward a patient is something of great importance !

Watches generally have become somewhat I think, superfluous. Most people have a clock at home, in the car, at work, on their phone, their computer. It is usually not difficult to dispense with a wrist watch.

As with any procedure or change with a patient, sometimes one single change as above, may bring about a spectacular reduction in a particular symptom or symptoms. At times a patient may remark that they have not experienced any positive change and yet that one change or intervention may be an essential part within a collection of changes necessary to bring about a desired result! The removal of jewellery is at the very least a simple measure and of no expense bar that of a patients sense of aesthetics or emotional significance.

SPINE / MUSCLE / SPORT

The first thing I would say here is that a healthy body, proper functioning of metabolic systems, organs, glands, nervous system, is essential for good athletic performance. What is happening internally will very much display or reflect upon muscle and joint function !

To properly assess physical ability and capacity for activity, the examination of muscle function is quite patently essential. Part of my undergraduate training covered the manual testing required to assess strength, power and function of skeletal muscles. It would seem obvious that we require strength in our muscles for daily activity and especially for adequate performance in sport, as such, detailed and thorough testing of muscles is indispensable.

With this in mind I pursued further postgraduate study of manual muscle testing predominantly via the ICAK (International College of Applied Kinesiology). This was of tremendous value in utilising basic theory that put forth that muscles will be influenced by the function of the spine, lymphatic drainage, quality of the blood, organs, glands, neurological, emotional, mental factors.

The essence here was that if I was to adjust a spinal vertebra there also existed the capacity to reduce imbalances in muscles that had contributed to the restriction of that bony joint. In the case where a joint was "stiff" there is the capacity to loosen surrounding muscles by addressing the causes of that muscle dysfunction as such by improving internal or organic and glandular function. Similarly an unstable or excessively mobile joint could be strengthened. In a fashion our nervous system could be pictured as a hand that operates a puppet and yet our bodies systems, glands, organs, metabolism, care for or "feeds" that nervous system. Therefore it is possible to "adjust" a joint by other means, that is, by working on internal systems.

What became a quantum step for me, was a postgraduate course presented by Michael Allen (see chapter 2). His own work (and I think somewhat brilliant!) and to a degree I surmise, springing from courses presented by Frederick Carrick, demonstrated the value of assessing muscle function to see or literally to, manually feel wether those muscles not only switch on or "facilitate" properly, switch off or " inhibit" properly, yet also that they do so at the appropriate time and position.

A simple description or illustration of the above would be for example that say a footballer with a hamstring strain may have that strain as a result of that hamstring muscle being unable to "switch off". Hence, as say his right leg goes forward the right hamstring muscle is respectively strained in part due to its lack of ability to lengthen sufficiently and of course if of a given level of severity, fatigue, or repetition, the muscle, its fascia or ligamentous structures therefore may rupture or tear.

Of course a similar strain may occur if the muscle was primarily "weak". The muscle may also receive and be capable of responding to signals to switch on and off yet may sustain additional influences so that those on's and off's do not occur at the required time or appropriate position and so again a resultant injury occurs.

By way of analogy, a dysfunctional set of muscles may behave as if the driver of a motor vehicle would press the accelerator pedal at an inappropriate time in preference to applying the brake or vice versa. This may be a poor form of driving a car, yet with regard to our physical body it is very likely to lead to muscle and joint strain or injury.

Within my own practice as a means to address muscle or spinal function I do consider the application where necessary of all factors discussed within this text. Though in looking for a practitioner who may be able to provide the required physical or clinical work the reader may find help in searching practitioners that have some qualification within the discipline of Applied Kinesiology and or those that have studied within the auspices of the Carrick Institute.

D N A

The explanation below is primarily to assist a patient to have a greater understanding with respect to how their body works. I believe it is worthwhile to demystify the subjects of health and illness as best I can so that this may offer some degree of comfort or reassurance. Also that a patient is often more likely with a higher level of understanding to feel a more positive motivation to make changes that may assist them. Most of the chapters within this book are along similar lines though this one is somewhat more specific and at the core of our biochemical function.

Your DNA, that is, deoxyribose nuclei acid doesn't just sit in your body's cells or cell nuclei waiting for you to be reproductive, produce an egg or sperm, i.e. have a child.

Your DNA is the blueprint which is copied so as to run your body, to run your metabolism i.e. to run your physical, mental and emotional life.

I write the following as a simple explanation. When your body wants to make something, a brain chemical (neurotransmitter), a ligament, a fat, energy, a hormone, it will unravel a segment or segments of DNA (a gene) and copy it into the form of RNA (ribonucleic acid). DNA is double strand molecule, RNA a single strand.

The RNA strand is passed out of the cell nucleus into the body of the cell (cytoplasm) and "read" on a ribosome. In simple terms you could think of a ribosome like a tape reader that "reads" the RNA segments which contain a "code" for specific amino acids.

There are roughly twenty amino acids and in this process and they carried on what are called t RNA or transfer RNA molecules.

The ribosome "reads" the RNA, and then "collects" and adds together a chain or string of amino acids to make a special protein (a large protein) called an enzyme.

These enzymes are specific to each gene. The enzyme is usually "switched on" by attaching a "vitamin" and a "mineral" obtained from our food.

This enzyme is if you like as if it were a little worker, or workers that will take a substance from our food, for one by example, cholesterol, and convert it in stages into a hormone (a steroid hormone). You could think of a steroid hormone as if it were like a letter or parcel in the mail. Whereas you could "picture" nerves or neural signals as if they were telephone lines or telephone messages. As such both of the above provide a means of communication within the body.

A steroid hormone, for example oestrogen will effect menstruation or testosterone for example to effect "male" characteristics.

If we sustain nutritional deficiencies or excesses within our bodies then our ability to make what we need to be healthy is compromised. If we carry segments of DNA or RNA from infections then we will make material which we don't need i.e. an autotoxic process, if I can term that, "an automatic toxicity". In essence what is TOXIC is what our body doesn't need or is unable to use or is too much of what we do need or use.

A simple explanation of how food could affect our DNA function is as follows. We make enzymes constantly or almost so.

To make an enzyme our systems have to find one of from a selection of twenty amino acids each time a segment of code is read which matches the gene code for that specific or required amino acid and do so each fraction of a second. The amino acids are attached to what is called transfer RNA which is like a carrier and added in sequence so as to make a required enzyme.

If we have a reasonably even supply or distribution or required levels of each amino acid, the ribosome then has if you like to find one friend at a party of twenty people. If we eat too much of a particular food, especially one of which that we may not be well suited, there may be as a result, excesses of a particular or individual amino acids.

This could be for example that there is the presence of far too much of one or two or three amino acids. As such our "ribosome" has to "find" one friend at a party of say sixty people. And thus the ribosome's speed of producing what we need slows down. Therefore we may as a result, heal more slowly, have less energy and not detoxify ourselves so readily nor have the requisite ability to deal with injurious or infectious processes.

We have metabolic systems that repair sites of damage to our DNA, as such, thousands of "repairs" daily, that is as an ongoing basis. We are also constantly making new cells and these new cells require a full complement or set of chromosomes (DNA). Our DNA is made from so called "bases", or purines and pyrimidine's. I consider that if we are eating foods and combinations of foods that provide a required bias of these "bases" that we are then more able to properly repair our DNA and to manufacture new cells with a healthy or with a healthier genetic complement. This is somewhat a radical idea and yet, if you consider the following.

Any manufacturing or building process if it is to be quick, efficient and able to produce the desired end result or product it will require the ready availability and relative numbers of the required constituent parts. For example it may be a slow process to build a motor vehicle if the manufacturer has an overwhelming glut of wheels and a poor supply or absence of the availability of engines.

Similarly with the production of nerve cell membranes, if we have an overwhelming excess of say oils of an eight carbon chain length and a significant deficiency of say ten carbon chain oils, then we are likely to produce an undesirable and dysfunctional cell or worse, no new cell at all.

I have outlined the above to emphasise what I believe is such an essential part of dealing with any "health" condition, that is to take very careful consideration of what food we eat, in what combination and as to how it is prepared. In essence I believe that with the careful and advised consideration of what we eat, that it is possible to alter our own or personal genetic constitution so as to have a better or greater level of health!

MENTAL EMOTIONAL

I believe that mental or emotional conditions can be altered with simple nutritional means. Yet with any such case various aspects need to be considered as the following,

- ➢ Biochemical disturbance
- ➢ Fatigue
- ➢ Environmental factors
- ➢ Situational considerations
- ➢ Beliefs or thought patterns, spiritual or philosophical perspectives

As previously with any condition it is essential to identify contributing or causative factors. Some of the most spectacular changes I have seen in a patient's mental emotional wellbeing or sense of feeling has been with utilising changes in consumption of food and the use of minerals, especially though by altering a patient's consumption of fats and oils. I would like to qualify the above somewhat in that I have had found for myself the experience and benefit, very much so of courses, so called spiritual, mental, emotional, "personal" development courses that have been so very valuable. Yet as with much of what I am writing here and have written within this book the bias is almost entirely toward physical considerations. Though as an aside I would add to this, it is said that discretion is the better part of valour, maybe it is that honesty is indispensable and with that, discretion is an essential part of openness.

To go on, a basic illustration of a simple nerve cell is I believe useful here, they are of course our means to enable experience and thinking. Cells within the body may be relatively flat e.g. skin cells or with various glands or organs, roughly round, though nerve cells are generally different.

A nerve cell in a basic form has a cell body containing the cell nucleus which then houses the chromosomes or DNA. Usually outgrowing from that cell body we have DENDRITES which may be seen as protruding branches or fingers. These dendrites connect with parts of other incoming or communicating nerves. The inputs to that cell are processed or summated and then the nerve cell "decides" whether or not to pass on a signal to another nerve cell or nerves, a muscle or a gland for example.

A nerve passes a signal via a short or long thin extension from itself which is referred to or called, an AXON. A signal travels up or down or across the brain or spinal cord or body to meet or "talk" to another nerve or tissue at a "SYNAPSE". With the appropriate signal having travelled down the axon, vesicles of a NEUROTRANSMITTER i.e. a brain chemical, will emit from the nerve terminal into the SYNAPTIC CLEFT i.e. the space between the two nerves.

The neurotransmitter then "meets" or attaches to the receiving cells receptors. The effect is to cause the receiving cell to either tend to switch on or switch off. This is somewhat like a computer which "talks" in BINARY NUMBERS i.e. zero's and one's which equates to either an on or an off.

As with any cell, the nerve cell has a "skin" or cell MEMBRANE which contains a large proportion of fats and oils.

Of all the potential dietary changes I have been able to use, the most satisfactory and startling changes I have seen with " mental / emotional" conditions have most often come from the following. Either using a roughage to help eliminate or exit from the body, "old" fats and oils or by removing, introducing or reintroducing a particular fat or oil into the diet. Specifically and as somewhat outlined in the above (DNA), a nerve will perform much better or more "happily" if it contains the appropriate fats or oils. Not uncommonly the simplest change has been to temporarily remove from the diet a cooking oil or salad dressing oil that the patient may have been using for a long time, i.e. for many years.

I will provide here for illustration, two examples. Four years ago I had noticed that a colleague of mine was not or did not seem her normal self. I said to her "you don't seem so happy", she appeared to be carrying a "black cloud", rather than her usual happy or ebullient self. She related to me that she had felt for quite a number of weeks, tired or angry, irritated. One aspect of the subsequent examination that I employed with her was to use a form of testing nerve cell ions, the ions listed as listed below.

➢ Calcium (++)
➢ Sodium (+)
➢ Potassium (+)
➢ Chloride (−)

As a nerve cell allows ions having a positive charge to pass into the inside of the AXON "tube", it will progress toward a point where the change in electrical potential difference or flow of ions will cause that nerve cell to "fire". An "electrical flow" then passes down the axon and then acts upon the end terminal of the nerve i.e. its destination and thus neurotransmitters are emitted, which pass across the synapse to the receptor cell, and so a signal has been sent and received.

The patient appeared, if I could say, upon testing, 'sensitive' to chloride ions. The chloride ion has a negative charge within this "environment" and so when a sufficient accumulation of negative charge enters the cell and or in addition, positive charge pumped out, the nerve is then more likely not to fire or to remain "at rest". The approach to testing the "negative chloride ions" as such demonstrated a "response" to the neurotransmitter , SEROTONIN. With healthy levels of serotonin, in general we are more inclined to feel well or happy.

As a theory, if we have too much or too little of a particular fat or oil then nerve cell membranes may have a sufficiently "altered resistance" and so be more likely or less likely to fire. Or in other terms, too " leaky" or too " impervious" to a particular ion or ions.

What appeared to negate this "negative" response was with the use of a simple cooking oil. The patient attained the required oil, and took three or four "swigs". Within an hour or so, she related to me that she felt that the 'blackness' had gone and a feeling of happiness had come as if she had drunk half a bottle of champagne. Please note, I like this example though it is not always that such a rapid response is achievable. Also that, there is no one single fat or oil which will produce such a change in every case. Most often it is that detailed examination and testing is required to determine a patient's specific need. On the other hand occasionally a patient will simply recognise that they have consumed large amounts of a particular fat or oil or food over a long period of time, change that and so experience some desired improvement in the way they feel.

The effect of what would appear to be a deficiency of a particular oil or oils within serotonin pathways could be seen as having caused a membrane dysfunction of sufficient degree so to allow a bias toward those nerves not firing or not firing as much as required and hence low serotonin levels and the experience of what would be called depression.

That is the dysfunctional membranes may well have allowed excessively raised chloride (-) ion concentrations within the nerve axon and so reduced the nerve's capacity to reach a firing threshold and thus a resultant deficiency in either the production and or release of serotonin.

A second case, a fellow in his early sixties, related to me that he had begun to experience during the day, visions or memories of a time, earlier in his life which he had found to be and was, terribly upsetting. He was also having a similar experience in the form of nightmares. The major change that I suggested was that he would undertake was to remove the consumption of canola oil from his diet. Please note that this advice was given only after employing a rather complex examination or convoluted series of tests and importantly, listening to what he had to say. One point that he made upon questioning i.e. "taking a history" was that for many years he had used a large volume, a table spoon of canola oil in the evenings to cook his dinner. This may seem a trivial point though sometimes a patient will mention something which could sound as if it were of little importance and yet be of a critical significance !

After a period of three days of having not used the canola oil, he related to me that the condition he had been experiencing was gone and that he had returned to a feeling of being happy.

Will exclusion or inclusion of a fat or oil within a patient's diet change all "mental" / "emotional" conditions? I would say not, yet once a specific excess or deficiency has been identified it can be to change that, a very useful therapeutic intervention.

The most common mineral deficiency I would see or perceive in practice, is a deficiency of IODINE. If you keep in mind, again this may well be significantly a facet of my practice location and the inherent genetic bias of the patient's that consult me.

To say for example if working in Mexico or Norway, if I did a see certain deficiencies with people living in those environments and with the inherent genetic makeup which they have, the above perceived deficiency of iodine may well be not be present.

In addition to iodine it is in my experience again commonly to see a deficiency of MAGNESIUM in patient's. A point to make here is that I would often see not only a deficiency of magnesium but also a distortion of the relative DISTRIBUTION of both MAGNESIUM and CALCIUM within a patient. As such I have developed approaches to address this, in part dealing with low grade infections, altering the diet and especially in so aiming at what may be a "healthy level of FLUORIDE in the body, see chapter 7.

With regard to magnesium I do not often hear mention of it either in lay conversation nor read of it commonly in the written media and yet it could be argued to be the most abundantly used or important mineral within our biochemistry. We very much require magnesium to produce energy, to make most of our vitamins work, to relax our muscles for example. Low levels of magnesium or poor distribution of magnesium and we will then tend toward a tired body, a tired brain. As iron may "compete" with iodine so magnesium may "compete" with calcium.

At least within Australia there is a relative tendency toward a high consumption of red meat and a high consumption of dairy food. The former tending to confer relatively high levels of iron and the latter toward high levels of calcium. As such I believe what is consistent with the above is that I very rarely supplement a patient with iron or calcium irrespective of what conventional thought or testing may dictate. Patient's that I have seen and that I have considered to be sustaining an excess of iron often have a propensity toward excessive inflammation and fatigue. Similarly a patient who would seem to be low in magnesium and retaining an excess of calcium are often predisposed to cramp and fatigue.

Returning to iodine, as before, I see it as a common deficit. It is not uncommon a patient (as previous, most of my patients are female) would report that they had had a feeling of being "teary". That is that they felt very emotionally sensitive, very prone to burst into tears. Often to treat this they would be advised to apply a small amount, roughly half a handful of proprietary" Betadine", to wet skin after a shower. Again not all "teary" or emotionally sensitive persons have an iodine deficit, yet it can be when a deficiency is present, a very quick effective treatment to simply apply a solution as a source of iodine so as to correct that deficiency and derive a positive result, often very rapidly. You would only use iodine though upon the advice of a qualified practitioner. In this regard a medical practitioner may use blood tests to determine a patient's iodine status and with respect to alternative health care practitioners some will consider that a patient is not deficient if a solution of iodine applied to the skin does not diminish in colour within a few hours of application.

Conversely if iodine is applied and the colour disappears rapidly some would consider the patient to be iodine deficient.

Why iodine? Firstly in general the consumption of red meat is at least where I live, of a relatively high level. An excess of iron in the diet creates in a manner of speaking a "competition" with iodine. That is to say they are somewhat opposed or antagonistic. Secondly, there is in the patients that I see, commonly a relatively low consumption of salt. The use of small amounts of sea salt or as I would often suggest "Himalayan" rock salt (both a source of iodine) and a lower consumption of red meat tends to be a sufficient change with patients to produce a better balance within their biochemistry between levels of iron and iodine.

Iodine is required to make the two major thyroid hormones. Thyroxin is referred to as T4. T4, that is T for thyroid and or T for tyrosine, T4 contains four "iodine" atoms. And T3 which is the more potent of the two contains three iodine atoms.

Here is what I believe a very common aspect with respect to mental / emotional conditions and that is the presence of fatigue or metabolic fatigue within a person's nervous system. With a deficiency of iodine there will be a tendency toward low levels of thyroid hormones and as a result of an insufficiency of energy production. Similarly, a deficiency of healthy fats and oils, and an excess of calcium within the nervous system will contribute to a sense of fatigue and if of enough significance be a cause of mental or emotional distress. In the first example energy production is low whereas in the second example there is a fatigue via too rapid a loss of energy.

I have in years past commonly used minerals of course other than iodine for example zinc or manganese and been able to achieve worthwhile responses. I have also made effective use of vitamins and or activated vitamins (coenzymes) as part of a therapeutic approach. Yet for quite a few years now with alteration of diet, home environment, personal hygiene, it is now rare for me to find those requirements. One common exception though would be and quite commonly seen is a deficiency of coenzyme Q10 (ubiquinone). Coenzyme Q10 is essential for the production of energy in the body and for healthy cardiac (heart) function. As an addition in my own experience it may also seem to have some important functions or effects within the immune system.

Some patients will demonstrate a response to a form of "testing" their nervous system to see if it would appear that they have some adverse response to the substance, GLUCOSAMINE. Please note that this section is along similar lines to that which is discussed in chapter 4. Glucosamine sulphate is the gelatinous hydrophilic (water loving) material generally present in CARTILAGE within our bodies joints. Our brain, our nervous system uses a many times greater amount of GLUCOSE as would be used by other tissues. Some of our neurotransmitters are amino acids or similar to amino acids, as the following four examples.

> Taurine
> Glycine
> Serine
> Glutamine

It would appear to me that upon using various forms of testing with a patient that has a level of dysfunction, there may exist an abnormal process of combining glucose with and an "amino acid" neurotransmitter. Thus in theory the possibility exists that at the terminal end of a nerve axon, deposits of glucosamine or a glucosamine like material could accumulate. Being a gelatinous like substance, it may then act to prevent or limit the normal transmission of neurotransmitter vesicles into the synaptic cleft so that signals may then as a result be poorly transferred to an adjoining nerve or nerves.

The most direct means to alter that dysfunction may simply be to address a patient's intake of sugars, and carbohydrates and a change in the type and amount of protein that they consume.

Primarily to alter protein intake, it would be most common to change the consumption of animal protein, beef, lamb and chicken. The most frequent change I would make in practice to alter protein intake is to limit the overall volume of animal protein commonly to reduce the intake of chicken and substitute with turkey.

Of course most foods have some level of protein content and so the above "gelatine phenomena", in theory, may respond in a positive way to an alteration of the intake of a variety of foods, vegetables, fruit, grains or beans.

BRIEF NOTES

A PRACTITIONER

My preference with a practitioner is to find one who is well qualified, caring, kind, considerate, empathic and willing to spend sufficient time. To be thorough in both the examination and treatment of a patient is an essential thing and something that takes time. Importantly and very much so with taking an oral history, that is asking the patient questions in detail, listening, hearing with a view to gaining an understanding of the patient, their complaint and causative factors of such. Within my own practice a patient being seen for the first time would have an appointment lasting approximately one hour. Subsequent visits range between thirty to sixty minutes. Time that a practitioner takes to examine thoroughly and with the use of a variety of means and constantly review a patient for me is an essential requirement.

At a high level with any sport a coach is required if one is to do well. Health I believe is little different, do your own work, educate yourself and find a practitioner that you like and trust.

SLEEP

It is said that being unable to sleep is the worst thing. Probably not quite the worst of human experiences, yet being able to sleep well is so very important. We make energy in our bodies for activity, to maintain a sufficient temperature, healing, repair, detoxification and elimination. With a lack of sleep we do not tend to heal so well. My own experience is that both pharmaceutical and herbal or homeopathic medicines can work well to assist in cases of insomnia. It is possible to identify specific causes of insomnia yet in general terms the healthier a patient is then the more likely they are to sleep well.

At times in a conversation with respect to sleep I would hear a standard response for example, "If you can't sleep you need MELATONIN". In reality a patient would likely, only need to supplement melatonin if they had a deficiency of that substance. Finding the cause and causes, removing them, providing required nutrition is I believe very important and often some form of physical intervention is useful.

Rest I suppose is somewhat a partner of sleep. If unable to sleep well, at least to have more rest can be a help. Certainly holidays, a change of scenery can with some patients make an important difference.

Some fifteen years ago a patient telephoned to speak to me regarding his wife. She was bedridden with severe back pain, migraine, was depressed and substantially overweight. I recommended that he would take her to a naturopath. The naturopaths approach was generally to put patients on an intake of organic fruit and vegetable juices. In addition and in my own experience patients were encouraged to sleep for most of the day and night. In sleeping, resting and using juices for nutrition, as they require less energy for digestion, a far greater level of energy was available for healing, detoxification and elimination.

The fellow's wife I believe stayed for about twelve days. I saw her three weeks after she had returned. She had no remaining symptoms nor illness and for a thirty year old woman she looked to me almost like a school girl, such was her level of improvement.

Specificity is paramount with any patient and as such a patient who is somewhat fatigued may respond very well to simply altering their normal routine where possible so as to gain more sleep or more rest !

COLOUR

You can change nervous system and biochemical function with colour! Even though colour can be a useful tool I believe to a large extent most people's preference either conscious or subconscious in their use and selection of colour is often good enough.

I will occasionally have a patient look at a particular colour as therapeutic exercise, include or exclude a colour either in either their clothing or home or work environments. Occasionally a patient will benefit from for example changing the tint of either prescription eyewear or sunglasses.

An interesting observation is that often if a patient demonstrates an adverse response to a particular colour upon some form of testing, then a food of similar colour may also seem to have an adverse effect upon them.

Occasionally the reverse is true, where there is a colour that appears to provide an improvement in some neurological function, the patient may respond well to eating a food of similar colour.

We are adapted in genetic terms to deal with light, quite obviously for example a native African has very dark skin, a Norwegian having skin which is "fair", very pale in colour. As such in some cases I will test a patient so as to look for responses to basic colours, including black.

There may be some benefit for a patient to eat at times food which has a very dark if not a black colour. If as humans we may have "black" skin to protect against excess radiation then it is likely that some vegetable use similar means.

Hence, as some foods may contain a high level of anti-oxidants, some foods may be useful in their capacity to absorb and so negate excess or adverse sources of radiation. For example, the skin of an Aubergine or black pepper may be useful in this respect.

RESEARCH

There is an enormous volume of work within refereed science journals which has addressed the study of human function. From this material often springs forth clinical work which would initially be "experimental", some of which in the fullness of time becomes conventionally accepted. As within the introduction of this book, my undergraduate studies and a great deal of my postgraduate study was and is of a conventional basis. Anything new has to begin with an idea, an observation, imagination. And so again much of what I have written is not relating to work that I undertook which is conventional but that which may be considered unusual or unique or unconventional.

With patients, what is learnt from research can be applied to great effect. Yet another perspective is that a great deal or research is carried out under what could be called BOXED DIAGNOSIS. For example some studies have shown an improvement of ARTHRITIC symptoms in those suffering that condition with the use of glucosamine sulphate supplementation.

If say one hundred subjects were trialled and on "average" there was demonstrated an improvement in those subjects over a period of time then a practitioner may think "we could try this approach and see how we go".

A diagnosis of arthritis, that is as a term 'arthros' for joint and 'itis' for inflammation. Thus a practitioner or researcher may work from the perspective of a 'box', as such "we have this diagnosis" and we have say, half a dozen "treatments" to choose from to apply with either a patient or research subject. The research in general, "averages" the results and as such when applying that research to a patient we can be left with only a probability of some success .What I consider here is in part a flaw within this "methodology" is that the causes of that " glucosamine" deficiency may well not have been addressed simply by providing supplementation. As a counterpoint a study may for example take, say one hundred "arthritic" patients and trial the effectiveness of using oral safflower oil as a remedy. It could be that perhaps one patient does very well and the rest have no noticeable benefit and thus the "research" conclusion is that in statistical terms the use of safflower as a treatment for arthritis is not beneficial. My point is to take and make use of formal research and in addition quite literally "research" each individual patient through both thorough and repetitive examination.

 Also to consider that once one treatment has been undertaken to consider that the patient is now different and thus continue to examine and re-examine them. Importantly, to do so, not only so as to assess the response or responses to treatment but in addition to see what new state of function they have acquired and how to further proceed.

AIDS / SEMEN

A healthy sperm or spermatozoa in semen is designed to find a female egg (ovum), penetrate the outer then nuclear membranes to provide half a genetic compliment. In its passage from the vagina to the egg, the sperm is somewhat protected from the females immune system.

To consider, is it that the following is possible. Is it that in a human being with either oral or rectal exposure to semen that there is then a suppression or deleterious alteration of immune function as a result of such exposure?

Also, is it possible that with individuals of poor health that a sperm cell could penetrate a cell other than an ovum and thus provide a cell with a very abnormal and potentially damaging genetic compliment?

It may be with that persons not having HIV or having exposure to that virus that avoiding oral or rectal semen may be a means to avoid some adverse health condition.

Furthermore, with respect to the consideration that low grade or pernicious infection plays a significant role in health, illness. If a male has low grade testicular infection or other genito-urinary infection there is the possibility that the sperm cell may acquire (as with a viral infection) genetic material from that infectious process. As such if the sperm cell nucleus contains either whole microbial organisms, a full genetic or partial genetic compliment from an infectious process there may exist the potential for non-fertilisation or genetic defects within the fertilised egg.

CHOLESTEROL

The following may be of interest with regard to cholesterol. This is not intended to influence or change advice with respect to how a patient is treated yet, as previous I prefer that patients have some understanding of what is happening in their bodies.

The majority would, I feel, believe that cholesterol is bad. Yet we either absorb or manufacture cholesterol and from that molecule make steroid hormones and vitamin D, also another molecule essential for energy production. Below as such a list of some examples

- Oestrogens
- Progesterone
- Testosterone
- Cortisol
- DHEA
- Aldosterone
- Vitamin D
- Co enzyme Q10

With regard to terminology LDL cholesterol is often referred to as bad. LDL refers to the Low Density Lipoprotein, i.e. a protein carrier to transport cholesterol to for example the brain or endocrine glands. HDL is a High Density Lipoprotein or so called good cholesterol. LDL transports cholesterol to where it is needed like a green grocer delivering vegetables and so in that view it is somewhat incorrect to refer to it as "bad".

HDL is the "dustman" taking out the waste, LDL and HDL are both required or both good. It is more correct that the used or converted or waste cholesterol would be referred to as" bad".

I consider that in many patients, cholesterol levels may not be the primary problem but what happens or what is happening to the cholesterol. For example, a patient with a chronic low grade infection, may acquire an excess or too rapid an oxidation of cholesterol. It is a concept that a practitioner may consider even though seemingly a radical idea, i.e. is my patient low in cholesterol and why?

As a standard, too much or too little of any nutrient can be a problem. As such some patients are low in cholesterol.

A deficiency of oestrogens and progesterone can confer menstrual dysfunction. Low testosterone can affect tissue strength and motivation for example, cortisol is required as an anti-inflammatory, vitamin D to affect calcium absorption, DHEA is a precursor for other steroids, androgens and some oestrogens.

ALDOSTERONE is required to excrete excess potassium. Cholesterol if limited can confer lower levels of Co Enzyme Q10 which is required for energy production.

Also as cholesterol is oxidised it is as such an antioxidant. Furthermore cholesterol can have positive effects with respect to our nerve cell membrane permeability.

A low or too low a level of cholesterol may then lead to a problematic nervous system as follows. High potassium can lead to nerves more likely to be excessively switched on. A "leaky" nerve cell membrane can require more energy to pump ions yet if Co Enzyme Q10is low and energy deficient we can have "tired" nerve cells or greater nerve cell death (trans neural degeneration)

DEODORANT

As with foot odour an axillary or underarm odour is in my experience often an indication of the presence of a low grade infectious process in the body. A patient with a low level of toxicity and the absence of infectious processes that are beyond the capacity of normal immune functions may rarely need to use a deodorant. As with the daily and multiple use of fluoride toothpaste it is possible to acquire an aluminium toxicity either locally under the arm or a varied distribution within the body. It is worthwhile in some cases to use an aluminium free deodorant or use in conjunction with, lesser frequently a commercial deodorant.

SHOES

I recall years ago reading the admonition, "never wear the same pair of shoes for two days in a row". It is not uncommon for a patient to remark that they are somewhat concerned if it is that their shoes or feet have an odour. An odour will often be from perspiration and as such, waste or toxic fluid and or not uncommonly a low grade infectious process.

As with the "dripping tap" idea, over a period of months or years, the inner lining of shoes may well accumulate a high concentration of toxic material. As such a patient runs a cycle of trying to eliminate waste from the soles of their feet and then REABSORBING this concentrated toxicity. Here it is a similar theme to an initially low grade irritation as with some jewellery or a "favourite" food over a period of time becoming a significant and adverse causation, providing an overload of toxicity. Many people would over a period of months or years put their feet into the same shoes on a daily basis without ever cleaning, protecting or replacing the inside lining. One would not imagine wearing a lining against their underarms for months or years in the same fashion.

As a simple means of intervention a patient may dispose of their old shoes and socks. I feel it has been of use to have patients insert a couple of layers of paper towel inside the shoes so as to absorb moisture and toxicity, also to limit that which would be absorbed into the shoe itself. Some patients have responded well to simply soaking their feet in a basin of warm water with half a teaspoon of dissolved Epsom salts. Others had found benefit in using proprietary foot detoxification pads. A far as culprits I consider running shoes likely the worst. Having three or four pairs of shoes does enable a patient to "air" those shoes that are not in use. In warm weather it is I consider useful to leave shoes in the sun so as to dry them out and to some extent limit the presence or growth of infectious processes.

Two cases by way of example, one patient, a fellow with a chronic urinary bladder complaint improved very much simply by "detoxifying" his feet and footwear. Another, a female patient related to me that if she regularly employed the use of a paper or tissue lining within her footwear that at the end of a working day she was much less likely to feel tired or "foggy in the head" or to feel an aching or soreness in her feet or legs. Where possible within the bounds of health and safety regulations I consider it is a worthwhile thing to at times throughout a day to remove ones shoes so as to "air" the shoes and feet.

Again here is not the cure for bladder conditions or fatigue yet it is part of the philosophy that reducing a patients toxic load, allowing the passage and exit of waste material, reducing the presence of infectious material, provides a greater ease from which a person may assist their physical body to function better, to heal itself.

A SYNOPSIS

This book is not presented and has not been written in a recipe format or a "this for that" approach. I am somewhat encouraging the reader to think for themselves to consider the environment in which they live and work and what they eat. To a degree I feel that the above has been for quite a long time part of a conventional "western" medical perspective and that is to be aware of hygiene and to eat well.

The material presented can be separated into two parts, that which the reader can do themselves and that which would essentially require professional help and guidance. Much of what I have written would be considered to be safe and simple as follows. The thorough cleaning of ones home environment, replacing old mattresses, bed linen, carpets, changing your shoes, the removal at least temporarily of earrings, jewellery all of which may sound trivial yet in my experience can be of such positive and significant benefit.

With regard to food, some that would be of good health may for example view their dietary habits and consider if they have been eating the same foods for long periods of time. As a basic approach within science it is often that to undertake some experiment that only one variable i.e. is changed at a time. In this the idea is if you change many things at once it may be impossible to tell what it was that made a difference. And so for example someone who had predominantly used a vegetable oil with which to cook may try another oil or bias their cooking toward baking boiling or steaming food to see if in doing so they come to notice a positive benefit. Or in a similar vein, if one had eaten for months or years the same vegetable, again Broccoli for example to stop for a week or two and see if there is some improvement in their sense of wellbeing

As a second part and as I have suggested or recommended to work with a qualified practitioner. Two, that is, patient and practitioner are more likely to be successful than one, that is the patient alone. That applies not only to someone with a specific health complaint or complaints but also and I think very much someone who feels well and would like to feel even better and or practice what may prevent the development of illness.

AUTHOR'S NOTE

It is not that the book is a history of my use of conventional means but as in the preliminary notes, a discussion of what generally may be viewed as radical ideas. If it is safe, quick and effective then that is a happy thing irrespective of the approach being seemingly unusual.

If it is that ideas or suggestions within this book does enable the reader, you or you and your practitioner to achieve a desired result, that would be a happy thing, I hope you go well!

As a final note, the work presented, the philosophies and perspectives developed here, came out of somewhat extreme circumstances and as it was written. I am and have been fortunate to love my work. Certainly a part of that is that some of the most delightful human beings that I have met have been and still are patients of mine. I am also very grateful and would like thank here, those patient's that have been so extraordinarily kind to me and so very helpful assisting in the production of this book.

www.ingramcontent.com/pod-product-compliance
Lightning Source LLC
Chambersburg PA
CBHW072248310526
45795CB00011B/421

* 9 7 8 1 4 9 3 6 4 1 2 0 8 *